ISBN: 9781073032105

7-Day
No-Cooking Diets

Tina Hudson, M.S.

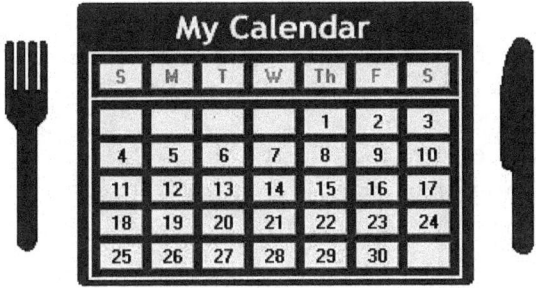

NoPaperPress™

<u>Note</u>: At publication, the off-the-shelf foods used in this book were widely available in most supermarkets. But food products come and go. So if there is a frozen entrée or soup selection in this diet that is out of stock, or that's been discontinued, or perhaps you don't like, or that you forgot to pick up while shopping, please substitute another food that has **<u>approximately</u>** the same caloric value and nutritional content. In this regard, many dieters have found the frozen foods and soups listed in the Appendices at the end of this book to be helpful.

CONTENTS

Most of us are busy – extremely busy struggling to balance career, family, finances, and then you need to make room for a personal life, for friends, for learning, for travel and the list goes on and on. Because you're so busy, you may neglect your health. You know you should lose weight. You want to lose weight but don't have the time to diet! Your life is just too hectic to plan and prepare elaborate low-calorie meals. That's where the 7-*Day No-Cooking Diets* can help.

When to Use 7-Day Diets

Maybe you've let your weight get out of control. So you decide to go on a diet. It doesn't matter what diet, or how much weight you want to lose. Your first move should be to go on the 7-*Day No-Cooking Diet,* lose a quick 3 to 5 pounds, and get on the right track. After the 7-day diet does its job you can switch to a longer-term diet. Our suggestion would be either the *30-Day Quick Diet* or the *90-Day Smart Diet*, both books come in a No-Cooking edition and both are published by NoPaperPress.

Maybe you're in weight maintenance mode but notice your weight creeping up. You want to stop the upward trend and lose a few pounds as well. Here's the perfect solution: Use the *7-Day No-Cooking Diet* to quickly lose those unwanted few pounds!

Understand that before you begin any weight loss program you should know your current health status. You also need to make sure your health will allow you to lower your caloric intake and increase your physical activity. A **medical checkup** is in order which may be as simple as a visit to a physician who is familiar with your medical history, or it may be a thorough physical exam. The physician conducting the medical exam should be made aware of and should approve the specific weight loss diet you're planning In particular, you should let your physician know that the 7-*Day No-Cooking Diet* **relies to a considerable degree on commercially processed foods** (frozen and microwaveable) – most of which have a relatively high salt (sodium) content.

What's in this Book?

This book actually contains **three 7-day no-cooking diets:** a 1500 Calorie diet, a 1200 Calorie diet and for even faster weight loss a 900-Calorie diet. All the diets have a meal plan (menu) for each and every day.

Which Calorie Level is for You?

Most **men** should choose the 1500-Calorie Diet. However, smaller men, inactive men and older men usually have more difficulty losing weight and therefore usually do better on the 1200-Calorie diet.

Most **women** should select the 1200-Calorie Diet. On the other hand, smaller women, inactive women and older women often find it harder to lose weight and, therefore, should consider the 900-Calorie Diet.

Understand, however, that due to the very low calorie level**, the 900-Calorie diet does not quite provide all the nutrients (protein, carbs and fat), micronutrients (vitamins and minerals) and fiber you need for good health.** Because it's a short term (7-Day) diet, however, this deficiency should not be a problem for most healthy people. Nevertheless, if you have any health problems or concerns, you definitely should avoid the 900-Calorie diet. Additionally, nearly everyone feels hungry on 900 Calories per day. It is not an easy diet to stay with.

How Much Weight Will You Lose?

Weight loss occurs when your food energy intake is less than the total energy you expend. This difference in calories is referred to as your calorie deficit. How much weight you lose depends on the magnitude of your calorie deficit. Physiologists have long known that to lose one pound requires a deficit of approximately 3500 Calories. Therefore, if a person's total calorie deficit over time is known, their weight loss over time can be calculated.

On the *7-Day No-Cooking Diet*, **most women lose 3 to 4 pounds** – depending on whether the 1200 or 900 Calorie diet is selected. Smaller women, older women and less active women will lose a bit less and larger women, younger women and more active women somewhat more.

On the *7-Day No-Cooking Diet*, **most men lose 4 to 5 pounds** – depending on whether the 1200 or 1500 Calorie diet is selected. Smaller men, older men and less active men will lose a bit less and larger men, younger men and more active men somewhat more.

Exactly how much weight you will lose depends on how much you weigh, your age and your activity level. Again, for the full story see *Weight Control - U.S. Edition* by Vincent Antonetti, Ph.D.

How to Use This Book

Depending on your size, your age and how active you are, select the diet calorie level that's right for you, either 900, 1200 or 1500 Calories per day.
  - **900-Calorie Diet** go to page 10.
  - **1200-Calorie Diet** go to page 18.
  - **1500-Calorie Diet** go to page 26.

Using the Daily Menus

Let's look at the Daily Menu for **Day 1 - 1200 Calorie**. Most of the menu is obvious and easily understood. To find the line item **Soup** go to page 43 **Appendix C**, first note that 110 Calories are allocated for the Day 1 soup. Then go to Appendix C (page 43) and find a list of soup in the diet. In Appendix C, scan the right-most column until you find 110 Calories. There are two soup selection to choose from.

Now let us move on to **Day 2 - 1200 Calorie**. To find the frozen entrée for Day 2 first note that the allotment for the frozen entrée is 300 Calories. Now go to page 44 **Appendix D**, which contains a list of frozen entrees arranged from lowest to highest calorie content. In Appendix D, scroll down until you find the 300 Calorie frozen entrees. The are nine to choose from.

900 Calorie Diet

Day 1 – 900 Calorie Meal Plan

BREAKFAST	Calories	Totals
Orange juice (½ cup)	50	
Wheaties (¾ cup) + ½ cup skim milk + ½ sliced banana	190	
Coffee (See Notes - page 40)	10	250 Cal
SNACK		
Coffee or tea	10	10 Cal
LUNCH		
Soup (Appendix C - page 43)	110	
Whole-grain bread (1 slice) (See page 40)	70	
Coffee or tea	10	190 Cal
SNACK		
Coffee or tea	10	10 Cal
DINNER		
Frozen Entrée (Appendix D - page 44)	200	
"Big-Bowl Salad" (See page 38 for ingredients)	150	
Water	0	440 Cal
SNACK		
Coffee or tea	10	10 Cal
		910 Cal

Day 2 – 900 Calorie Meal Plan

BREAKFAST	Calories	Totals
Fresh or frozen strawberries (½ cup)	25	
Kashi Go Lean Waffles (1)	75	
Light Syrup (1 Tbsp)	25	
Coffee	10	135 Cal
SNACK		
Coffee or tea	10	10 Cal
LUNCH		
Ham (2 oz) with mustard on 1 slice rye bread	220	
Fresh fruit in season (apple, peach, etc)	70	
Hot or iced tea	10	300 Cal
SNACK		
Yogurt (4 oz, non-fat, any flavor - see page 39)	60	60 Cal
DINNER		
Frozen Entrée (Appendix D - page 44)	220	
"Big-Bowl Salad" (See page 38 for ingredients)	150	
Water with lemon wedge	15	385 Cal
SNACK		
Coffee or tea	10	10 Cal
		900 Cal

Day 3 – 900 Calorie Meal Plan

BREAKFAST	Calories	Totals
Orange juice (½ cup)	50	
Scrambled egg (See Notes - page 40)	80	
Whole-grain toast (1 slice)	65	
Coffee	10	205 Cal
SNACK		
Coffee or tea	10	10 Cal
LUNCH		
Subway 6" (Turkey Breast, Cheese + veggies)*	230	
Yogurt (4 oz, non-fat, any flavor)	60	
Diet soda or water	0	290 Cal
* On half whole-grain roll		
SNACK		
Coffee or tea	10	10 Cal
DINNER		
Frozen Entrée (Appendix D - page 44**)**	230	
"Big-Bowl Salad"	150	
Water	0	380 Cal
SNACK		
Coffee or tea	10	10 Cal
		905 Cal

Day 4 – 900 Calorie Meal Plan

BREAKFAST	Calories	Totals
Cantaloupe (½ medium)	50	
Cheerios (1 cup) + ½ cup skim milk	160	
Coffee	10	220 Cal
SNACK		
Coffee or tea	10	10 Cal
LUNCH		
Cottage cheese (1 cup low fat)	180	
Fresh fruit in season (apple, plum, etc)	70	
Water	0	250 Cal
SNACK		
Coffee or tea	10	10 Cal
DINNER		
Frozen Entrée (Appendix D - page 44)	250	
"Big-Bowl Salad"	150	
Water	0	400 Cal
SNACK		
Coffee or tea	10	10 Cal
		900 Cal

Day 5 – 900 Calorie Meal Plan

BREAKFAST	Calories	Totals
Cantaloupe (½ medium)	50	
Fried egg	80	
Toasted raisin bread (1 slice)	75	
Coffee	10	215 Cal
SNACK		
Coffee or tea	10	10 Cal
LUNCH		
Chicken, Bacon Ranch*	270	
Coffee or tea	10	280 Cal
* Hot Pockets (wrap). If unavailable an equivalent food.		
SNACK		
Coffee or tea	10	10 Cal
DINNER		
Frozen Entrée (Appendix D - page 44)	200	
"Big-Bowl Salad"	150	
Water with lemon wedge	15	365 Cal
SNACK		
Coffee or tea	10	10 Cal
		900 Cal

Day 6 – 900 Calorie Meal Plan

BREAKFAST	Calories	Totals
Tomato juice (½ cup)	20	
Shredded Wheat (1 cup) + ½ cup skim milk	215	
Coffee	10	245 Cal
SNACK		
Coffee or tea	10	10 Cal
LUNCH		
Salad (3 oz canned tuna, 1 tsp Evoo, onions, celery)	175	
Small bunch of grapes	50	
Diet soda or water	0	225 Cal
SNACK		
Coffee or tea	10	10 Cal
DINNER		
Frozen Entrée (Appendix D - page 44)	250	
"Big-Bowl Salad"	150	
Water	0	400 Cal
SNACK		
Coffee or tea	10	10 Cal
		900 Cal

Day 7 – 900 Calorie Meal Plan

BREAKFAST	Calories	Totals
Orange juice (½ cup)	50	
Wheaties (¾ cup) + ½ cup skim milk + ½ banana	190	
Coffee	10	250 Cal
SNACK		
Coffee or tea	10	10 Cal
LUNCH		
Soup (Appendix C - page 43)	130	
String cheese (1 piece, any brand)*	80	
Coffee or tea	10	220 Cal
* Maximum of 80 Calories		
SNACK		
Coffee or tea	10	10 Cal
DINNER		
Frozen Entrée (Appendix D - page 44)	240	
"Big-Bowl Salad"	150	
Hot or iced tea	10	400 Cal
SNACK		
Coffee or tea	10	10 Cal
		895 Cal

1200 Calorie Diet

Day 1 – 1200 Calorie Meal Plan

BREAKFAST	Calories	Totals
Orange juice (½ cup)	50	
Wheaties (¾ cup) + ½ cup skim milk + ½ banana	190	
Coffee (See Notes - page 40)	10	250 Cal
SNACK		
Fresh fruit in season (apple, peach, etc)	70	
Coffee or tea	10	80 Cal
LUNCH		
Soup (Appendix C - page 43)	110	
Whole-grain bread (1 slice) (See page 40)	70	
Coffee or tea	10	190 Cal
SNACK		
Handful unsalted mixed nuts	100	
Coffee or tea	10	110 Cal
DINNER		
Frozen Entrée (Appendix D - page 44)	300	
"Big-Bowl Salad" (See page 38 for ingredients)	150	
Hot or iced tea	10	460Cal
SNACK		
Skinny Cow Low Fat Fudge Bar	100	
Coffee or tea	10	110 Cal
		1200 Cal

Day 2 – 1200 Calorie Meal Plan

BREAKFAST	Calories	Totals
Fresh or frozen strawberries (½ cup)	25	
Kashi Go Lean Waffles (2)	150	
Light Syrup (2 Tbsp)	50	
Coffee	10	235 Cal
SNACK		
Coffee or tea	10	10 Cal
LUNCH		
Ham (2 oz) with mustard on 2 slices rye bread	290	
Fresh fruit in season (apple, peach, etc)	70	
Coffee or tea	10	370 Cal
SNACK		
Yogurt (4 oz, non-fat, any flavor - see page 39)	60	60 Cal
DINNER		
Frozen Entrée (Appendix D - page 44)	220	
"Big-Bowl Salad" (See page 38 for ingredients)	150	
Hot or iced tea	10	380 Cal
SNACK		
Skinny Cow Ice Cream Sandwich	140	
Coffee or tea	10	150 Cal
		1205 Cal

Day 3 – 1200 Calorie Meal Plan

BREAKFAST	Calories	Totals
Grapefruit (½)	75	
Scrambled egg (See page 41)	80	
Whole-grain toast (1 slice)	70	
Coffee	10	235 Cal
SNACK		
Coffee or tea	10	10 Cal
LUNCH		
Subway 6" (Ham, Cheese +veggies)*	260	
Coffee or tea	10	270 Cal
* On half whole-grain roll		
SNACK		
Fresh fruit in season (pear, plum, etc)	70	
Coffee or tea	10	80 Cal
DINNER		
Frozen Entrée (Appendix D - page 44)	260	
"Big-Bowl Salad"	150	
Whole-grain bread (1 slice)	70	
Water with lemon wedge	15	495 Cal
SNACK		
Skinny Cow Low Fat Fudge Bar	100	
Coffee or tea	10	110 Cal
		1200 Cal

Day 4 – 1200 Calorie Meal Plan

BREAKFAST	Calories	Totals
Grapefruit (½)	75	
Cheerios (1 cup) + ½ cup skim milk	160	
Coffee	10	245 Cal
SNACK		
Coffee or tea	10	10 Cal
LUNCH		
Cottage cheese (1 cup low fat)	180	
Fresh fruit in season (apple, plum, etc)	70	
Small whole-grain roll	80	
Hot or iced tea	10	340 Cal
SNACK		
Coffee or tea	10	10 Cal
DINNER		
Frozen Entrée (Appendix D - page 44)	270	
"Big-Bowl Salad"	150	
Whole-grain bread (1 slice)	70	
Water	0	490 Cal
SNACK		
Handful unsalted mixed nuts	100	
Coffee or tea	10	110 Cal
		1205 Cal

Day 5 – 1200 Calorie Meal Plan

BREAKFAST	Calories	Totals
Cantaloupe (½ medium)	50	
Fried egg	80	
Toasted raisin bread (1 slice)	75	
Coffee	10	215 Cal
SNACK		
Banana (1 medium)	100	
Coffee or tea	10	110 Cal
LUNCH		
Salad (3 oz tuna, 1 tsp Evoo, onions & celery)	175	
Lettuce & tomato wedges	20	
Rye bread (1 slice)	65	
Diet soda or water	0	260 Cal
SNACK		
Yogurt (4 oz, non-fat, any flavor)	60	
Coffee or tea	10	70 Cal
DINNER		
Frozen Entrée (Appendix D - page 44)	210	
"Big-Bowl Salad"	150	
Fresh fruit in season (apple, peach, etc)	70	
Water with lemon wedge	15	445 Cal
SNACK		
Handful unsalted mixed nuts	100	100 Cal
		1200 Cal

Day 6 – 1200 Calorie Meal Plan

BREAKFAST	Calories	Totals
Tomato juice (½ cup)	20	
Shredded Wheat (1 cup) + ½ cup skim milk + ½ banana	265	
Coffee	10	295 Cal
SNACK		
Coffee or tea	10	10 Cal
LUNCH		
Chicken Pot Pie*	230	
Fresh fruit in season (apple, plum, etc)	70	
Diet soda or water	0	300 Cal
* Hot Pockets Wrap - if unavailable an equivalent food.		
SNACK		
Coffee or tea	10	10 Cal
DINNER		
Frozen Entrée (Appendix D - page 44)	260	
"Big-Bowl Salad"	150	
Whole-grain bread (1 slice)	70	
Water	0	480 Cal
SNACK		
Popcorn Mini Bag**	110	
Coffee or tea	10	120 Cal
**Such as Orville Redenbacher's Smart Pop		1205 Cal

Day 7 – 1200 Calorie Meal Plan

BREAKFAST	Calories	Totals
Orange juice (½ cup)	50	
Wheaties (¾ cup) + ½ cup skim milk + ½ banana	190	
Coffee	10	250 Cal
SNACK		
Coffee or tea	10	10 Cal
LUNCH		
Soup (Appendix C - page 43)	120	
String Cheese (1 piece, any brand)*	80	
Whole-grain bread (1 slice)	70	
Coffee or tea	10	280 Cal
* Maximum of 80 Calories		
SNACK		
Coffee or tea	10	10 Cal
DINNER		
Frozen Entrée (Appendix D - page 44)	300	
"Big-Bowl Salad"	150	
Fresh fruit in season (apple, peach, etc)	70	
Hot or iced tea	10	530 Cal
SNACK		
Popcorn Mini Bag	110	
Coffee or tea	10	120 Cal
		1200 Cal

1500 Calorie Diet

Day 1 – 1500 Calorie Meal Plan

BREAKFAST	Calories	Totals
Orange juice (½ cup)	50	
Wheaties (¾ cup) + ½ cup skim milk + ½ banana	190	
Whole-grain toast (1 slice) (See page 40)	70	
Coffee (Notes - page 40)	10	320 Cal
SNACK		
Fresh fruit in season (pear, plum, etc)	70	
Coffee or tea	10	80 Cal
LUNCH		
Soup (Appendix C - page 43)	110	
String cheese (1 piece, any brand)*	80	
Whole-grain bread (1 slice)	70	
Coffee or tea	10	270 Cal
* Maximum of 80 Calories		
SNACK		
Handful unsalted mixed nuts	100	
Coffee or tea	10	110 Cal
DINNER		
Frozen Entrée (Appendix D - page 44)	300	
"Big-Bowl Salad" (See page 38 for ingredients)	150	
Whole-grain bread (1 slice)	70	
Fresh fruit in season (apple, peach, etc)	70	
Hot or iced tea	10	600 Cal
SNACK		
Popcorn Mini Bag*	110	
Coffee or tea	10	120 Cal
*Such as Orville Redenbacher's Smart Pop		1500 Cal

Day 2 – 1500 Calorie Meal Plan

BREAKFAST	Calories	Totals
Fresh or frozen strawberries (½ cup)	25	
Kashi Go Lean Waffles (2)	150	
Morningstar Breakfast Sausage Links (2)	80	
Light Syrup (2 Tbsp)	50	
Coffee	10	315 Cal
SNACK		
Yogurt (4 oz, non-fat, any flavor - see page 39)	60	
Coffee or tea	10	70 Cal
LUNCH		
Ham (2 oz) with mustard on 2 slices rye bread	290	
Laughing Cow Light Cheese (1 wedge)	35	
Fresh fruit in season (apple, peach, etc)	70	
Coffee or tea	10	405 Cal
SNACK		
Handful unsalted mixed nuts	100	
Coffee or tea	10	110 Cal
DINNER		
Frozen Entrée (Appendix D - page 44)	220	
"Big-Bowl Salad" (See page 38 for ingredients)	150	
Whole-grain bread (1 slice)	70	
Hot or iced tea	10	450 Cal
SNACK		
Skinny Cow Ice Cream Sandwich	140	
Coffee or tea	10	150 Cal
		1500 Cal

Day 3 – 1500 Calorie Meal Plan

BREAKFAST	Calories	Totals
Grapefruit (½)	75	
Scrambled egg (See Notes - page 41)	80	
Turkey bacon (2 slices)	70	
Whole-grain toast (2 slices)	140	
Coffee	10	375 Cal
SNACK		
Yogurt (4 oz, non-fat, any flavor)	60	
Coffee or tea	10	70 Cal
LUNCH		
Salad (3 oz tuna, 1 tsp Evoo, onions & celery)	175	
Lettuce & tomato wedges	20	
Rye bread (1 slice)	65	
Fresh fruit in season (apple, plum, etc)	70	
Diet soda or water	0	330 Cal
SNACK		
Handful unsalted mixed nuts	100	
Coffee or tea	10	110 Cal
DINNER		
Frozen Entrée (Appendix D - page 44)	260	
"Big-Bowl Salad"	150	
Whole-grain bread (1 slice)	70	
Water with lemon wedge	15	495 Cal
SNACK		
Popcorn Mini Bag	110	
Coffee or tea	10	120 Cal
		1500 Cal

Day 4 – 1500 Calorie Meal Plan

BREAKFAST	Calories	Totals
Grapefruit (½)	75	
Cheerios (1 cup) + ½ cup skim milk + about 15 raisins*	190	
Coffee	10	275 Cal
SNACK		
Kashi TLC Crunchy Granola Bar	180	
Coffee or tea	10	190 Cal
LUNCH		
Cottage cheese (1 cup low fat)	180	
Fresh fruit in season (apple, peach, etc)	70	
Small whole-grain roll	80	
Hot or iced tea	10	340 Cal
SNACK		
Handful unsalted mixed nuts	100	
Coffee or tea	10	110 Cal
DINNER		
Frozen Entrée (Appendix D - page 44)	270	
"Big-Bowl Salad"	150	
Whole-grain bread (1 slice)	70	
Water with lemon section	15	505 Cal
SNACK		
Fresh fruit in season (apple, plum, etc)	70	
Coffee or tea	10	80 Cal
* See page 41 re substituting blueberries for raisins.		1500 Cal

Day 5 – 1500 Calorie Meal Plan

BREAKFAST	Calories	Totals
Cantaloupe (½ medium)	50	
Fried egg	80	
Toasted raisin bread (1 slice)	75	
Coffee	10	215 Cal
SNACK		
Yogurt (4 oz, non-fat, any flavor)	60	
Coffee or tea	10	70 Cal
LUNCH		
Soup (Appendix C - page 43)	280	
Whole-grain bread (1 slice)	70	
Banana (1 medium)	100	
Water	0	430 Cal
SNACK		
Fresh fruit in season (apple, plum, etc)	70	
Coffee or tea	10	80 Cal
DINNER		
Frozen Entrée (Appendix D - page 44)	210	
"Big-Bowl Salad"	150	
Fresh fruit in season (apple, peach, etc)	70	
Glass of wine (4 oz)	100	
Water with lemon wedge	15	555 Cal
SNACK		
Skinny Cow Ice Cream Sandwich	140	
Coffee or tea	10	150 Cal
		1500 Cal

Day 6 – 1500 Calorie Meal Plan

BREAKFAST	Calories	Totals
Tomato juice (½ cup)	20	
Shredded Wheat (1 cup) + ½ cup skim milk + ½ banana	265	
Coffee	10	295 Cal
SNACK		
Yogurt (4 oz, non-fat, any flavor)	60	
Coffee or tea	10	70 Cal
LUNCH		
Chicken Pot Pie*	230	
Fresh fruit in season (apple, peach, etc)	70	
Diet soda or water	0	300 Cal
* Hot Pockets Wrap - if unavailable an equivalent food.		
SNACK		
Handful unsalted mixed nuts	100	
Coffee or tea	10	110 Cal
DINNER		
Frozen Entrée (Appendix D - page 44)	260	
"Big-Bowl Salad"	150	
Whole-grain bread (1 slice)	70	
Fresh blueberries, cherries or grapes (1 cup)	100	
Water	0	580 Cal
SNACK		
Kashi TLC Chewy Granola Bar	140	
Coffee or tea	10	150 Cal
		1505 Cal

Day 7 – 1500 Calorie Meal Plan

BREAKFAST	Calories	Totals
Orange juice (½ cup)	50	
Wheat Chex (¾ cup) + ½ cup skim milk + ½ banana	250	
Coffee	10	310 Cal
SNACK		
Fresh fruit in season (apple, plum, etc)	70	
Coffee or tea	10	80 Cal
LUNCH		
Soup (Appendix C - page 43)	110	
String cheese (1 piece, any brand)	80	
Whole-grain bread (1 slice)	70	
Coffee or tea	10	270 Cal
SNACK		
Handful unsalted mixed nuts	100	
Coffee or tea	10	110 Cal
DINNER		
Frozen Entrée (Appendix D - page 44)	310	
"Big-Bowl Salad"	150	
Whole-grain bread (1 slice)	70	
Fresh fruit in season (apple, peach, etc)	70	
Hot or iced tea	10	610 Cal
SNACK		
Pop Popcorn Mini Bag	110	
Coffee or tea	10	120 Cal
		1500 Cal

Appendix A
Shopping Tips

No cooking doesn't mean no preparation! You will probably have to shop once a week. The following should help you prepare your shopping list.

First, understand that the problem with basing a meal plan on name-brand food items, such as a particular Lean Cuisine frozen entree, is that the item might not be available where you shop, or it may have been discontinued. What to do? That's where Appendices C and D in this book come in handy. Appendix C lists 19 name-brand soups in microwaveable bowls. Appendix D lists almost 150 name-brand frozen meals with their calorie count. Using these lists you should be able to find a substitute for the soup or frozen entree you can't find - a substitute that is based on the same food type, e.g., chicken, fish, or meat, and has the same approximate calorie count.

Substituting Foods

If there is a food listed in the diet you don't like, or perhaps that you forgot to pick up while shopping, you probably can exchange or substitute another food in its place – a technique used by dieticians. Exchanging a food listed in a diet for another food with approximately equal caloric value and nutritional content is the foundation of a successful long-term diet.

Substitution possibilities are almost endless but have to be done carefully. The easiest substitutions are those within the same food group, such as exchanging one vegetable variety for another, or a glass of milk for a cup of yogurt. More sophisticated exchanges cross food groups, for instance replacing 3½ ounces of turkey with a tablespoon of peanut butter spread on a piece of whole wheat bread. Both foods are complete proteins and both contain about 175 Calories. Refer to a good online calorie table to find calorie values. With some understanding and experience, you will be able to substitute foods called for in this diet with equal calorie foods from the same food group.

Another alternative is the following Food Substitution List that suggests substitutions for a variety of food items that appear in the daily meal plans. For example, Day 5 of the diet calls for half a cantaloupe for breakfast. But suppose cantaloupe is not in season, or just doesn't look good, or maybe it's too expensive, or you can't find it at your grocery, from the Food Substitution List you find that you may exchange a ½ cup of orange juice for half cantaloupe – both are in the fruit category and both contain about 50 Calories.

Light Syrup - Use any light syrup (25 Calories per Tbsp)
Big-Bowl Salad - Exchange with unlimited steamed greens (spinach, etc)
Cantaloupe (½) - Use ½ cup Orange juice
Cereal - Exchange with any other whole-grain cereal
Cottage Cheese (1 cup) - Two 8 oz glasses skim milk
Yogurt - Select 6 ounces skim milk
Eggs – Use Egg Beaters
Fresh fruit - ¾ cup canned fruit (no sugar added)
Frozen entrée - Substitute frozen entrée with same calories.
Grapefruit (½) - Choose an orange (medium)
Handful of Nuts - Popcorn Mini Bag
Kashi Chewy Granola Bar - Quaker Chewy Dipps Granola Bar
Kashi Go Lean Waffles - Eggo Nutri-Grain Whole Wheat Frozen Waffles
Hot Pockets Wraps - Lean Pockets Wraps
Morningstar Breakfast Sausage - Any breakfast sausage with comparable calories
String Cheese - Laughing Cow light cheese (2 wedges)
Popcorn - Use handful of mixed nuts
Raisin bread - Plain whole-grain bread
Skinny Cow Ice Cream Sandwich - Skinny Cow Low Fat Fudge Bar
Soup - Choose any soup with same calorie count
Whole-grain Bread - Vary bread type (whole wheat, rye, etc)
Wine (4 oz) - Instead select grapes (1 cup)

Finally, as a general rule, whenever you encounter a product on this diet, such as "Skinny Cow Ice Cream Sandwich" or "Kashi Go Lean Waffles," that has been discontinued or is out of stock, substitute another item of approximately equal caloric value and nutritional content. In other words find and substitute a different ice cream product or a different waffle brand.

Appendix B
7-Day Guidelines

Breakfast Guidelines

You've heard it before. It's important to start the day right and eat breakfast. **So try to allow time for breakfast before you rush off to work.** If need be do some preliminary preparation the night before such as setting up your coffee maker, deciding on and measuring the amount of cereal you will be eating, etc. Many busy people prepare breakfast at home and bring it to work in a plastic container. Do what you need to do – but don't skip breakfast!

In the *7-Day No-Cooking Diets,* you may substitute any wholesome **whole-grain cereal** for any specified cereal. For example, if you're not crazy about having Shredded Wheat for breakfast on Day 6, substitute Wheat Chex or Cheerios, etc. And if you don't like the fried egg called for on Day 5, have a hard-boiled egg or make a scrambled egg instead. Maybe the cantaloupe called for in the meal plan is not in season. No problem. Just replace the cantaloupe with a half cup of orange juice. For a more complete list of food substitutions and exchanges go to page 34.

Lunch Guidelines

On a *7-Day No-Cooking Diet,* lunch on most days will consist of either soup or a sandwich. For your convenience, soup choices have been limited to those sold in a microwaveable bowl. In fact, **unless otherwise stated, assume the soups specified in the 7-Day meal plans are microwaveable bowl versions.**

Soup: Appendix C (page 43) contains a list of soup selections that are perfect for busy adults on the go. Soup selections are from three of the leading producers of microwaveable soups (Campbell's, Healthy Choice and Progresso) and should be easily found in most supermarkets. All have been taste-tested by the authors and deemed acceptable to very good.

Feel free to substitute other soup brands you favor in place of those indicated – provided the type of soup and calorie counts are similar to those specified in the *7-Day No-Cooking Diet.* For example, the diet calls for Campbell's Tomato Soup (110 Calories). Notice in the previous example, the type of soup substituted was the same and the calorie count close.

Healthy Foods: Since 1994 the FDA has allowed the term "healthy" to be placed on the labels of certain foods that are comparatively low in total and saturated fat, that meet limits for sodium and cholesterol, and that contain some other micronutrients. **Note that most commercial soups are loaded with salt (sodium), the exceptions being Campbell's Healthy Request® soups, Healthy Choice soups and some canned Progresso lower-sodium soups** (not listed in Appendix C).

Warm Weather Substitutions: On warm and especially very hot days, you may want to substitute a sandwich, a tuna salad or a salmon salad if soup is on the menu.

Dinner Guidelines

Most of the dinners in the *7-Day No-Cooking Diet* are centered on a frozen entrée from one of the three leading manufacturers (Healthy Choice, Lean Cuisine and Weight Watcher's Smart Ones) and again should be easy to find at your local supermarket. Once more, all have been taste-tested by the authors and judged acceptable to very good.

About Frozen Foods

Busy families, singles, older people, and office workers alike enjoy the simplicity and convenience of a frozen meal. Many offices have an employee freezer jammed with all kinds frozen meals, which get zapped in a microwave for a quick, portable, portion controlled, and relatively inexpensive lunch.

As mentioned earlier, a high percentage of *7-Day No-Cooking Diet* dinners are based on frozen entrees. The specified frozen entrees, as well as others, are listed in **Appendix D,** pages 44 to 49.

In some instances, frozen may actually be better than fresh, because if you keep fresh fruit and vegetables in your fridge for a long time, they lose some of their nutritional value. Whereas, frozen fruits and vegetables are usually processed and packaged within hours of being picked. And the freezing process does not destroy nutrients. So buying frozen and then defrosting when you want the fruit or vegetable can actually retain more nutrients.

According to the U.S. Department of Agriculture, food stored continuously at 0 °F is safe to eat. Freezing keeps food safe and preserves food for extended periods because it prevents the growth of microorganisms that cause both food spoilage and food-borne illness.

Because freezing keeps food safe almost indefinitely, recommended freezer storage times are to preserve quality (taste, etc) of food, not the safety or nutritional value. **The quality of frozen dinners or entrees in a freezer at 0 °F is maintained for 3 to 4 months**.

Use an appliance thermometer to check your freezer's temperature. If a refrigerator's freezer can't maintain 0° F or if the freezer door is opened frequently, only use it for short-term food storage, and eat those foods as soon as possible for best quality. Use a free-standing freezer set at 0° F or below for long-term storage of frozen foods.

If there is a power outage, or if your freezer fails, or if the freezer door is left ajar by mistake, the food may still be safe to use. As long as a freezer with its door ajar continues to run, to cool, the foods should stay safe overnight. If a repairman is on the way or it appears the power will be restored soon, just keep your freezer door closed. A freezer full of food will usually keep about two days if the door is kept shut; a half-full freezer will last about a day. But the freezing compartment of a refrigerator may not keep foods frozen as long. (If the freezer is not full, group packages together to help maintain their low temperature.) During a power failure, you may want to put dry ice, a block or bags of ice in the freezer, o transfer foods to a friend's freezer until power is restored. Again, use an appliance thermometer to monitor the temperature. To determine the safety of foods when the power goes on, check their condition and temperature. If food is partly frozen, still has ice crystals, or is as cold as if it were in a refrigerator (40°F), it is usually safe to refreeze or use. It's not necessary to cook raw foods before refreezing. **If in doubt, however, always discard the food. And always discard frozen food whose temperature has exceeded 40°F for more than two hours.**

Sodium Problem

Sodium and sodium chloride (salt) normally occur in small quantities in many natural foods. People also add salt during food preparation and to the food they eat. But the average sodium intake for American adults is about 3,400 mg daily – more than 1,000 mg higher than the upper limit of 2,400 mg per day recommended by the U.S. Department of Health and Human Services and the Department of Agriculture Dietary Guidelines. (Note that one level teaspoon of salt contains about 2,300 mg of sodium.)

Although sodium plays an important role in your body, many studies have demonstrated that high sodium intake results in excessive water retention which causes blood volume to expand which in turn raises blood pressure. Moreover, some people are more sensitive to the effects of sodium than are others. These sodium-sensitive people retain sodium more easily. If you're in that group, extra sodium in your diet increases your chance of developing high blood pressure, a condition that can lead to cardiovascular and kidney diseases. Individuals who have high blood pressure and who are also salt sensitive are frequently advised to limit their sodium intake even further.

The downside to commercially prepared frozen entrees is that they frequently are loaded with too much salt (sodium). Be aware that, because of the relatively high sodium content of the frozen dinners and microwaveable soups, **the *7-Day No-Cooking Diets* may not be appropriate for everyone.**

In fact, you should have a medical checkup before beginning this weight loss diet. And let your physician know that the *7-Day No-Cooking Diets* rely to a large degree on commercially processed convenience foods (frozen and microwaveable) – many of which have a relatively high salt (sodium) content.

Big-Bowl Salad Every Day

Yet another problem with nearly all frozen entrees is that they don't contain enough veggies. The solution is to have a "Big-Bowl Salad" at dinnertime with your frozen entrée. A typical "Big-Bowl Salad" is shown on the following page.

To prepare a "Big-Bowl Salad" start with a relatively large soup bowl (with a volume of at least 24 ounces, or 3 cups). Add about 1½ cups of either green leaf lettuce, Romaine lettuce or a mix. Then add, as desired, veggies such as broccoli, celery, cucumber, onion, peppers, radish, spinach, tomato, or watercress, to make up the remaining 1½ cups, for a total of 3 cups. This vegetable combination will, on average, total about 100 Calories. You will be eating a "Big-Bowl Salad" every day at dinnertime. Remember that variety is the key to a nutritious diet. So be sure to vary the ingredients of the salad.

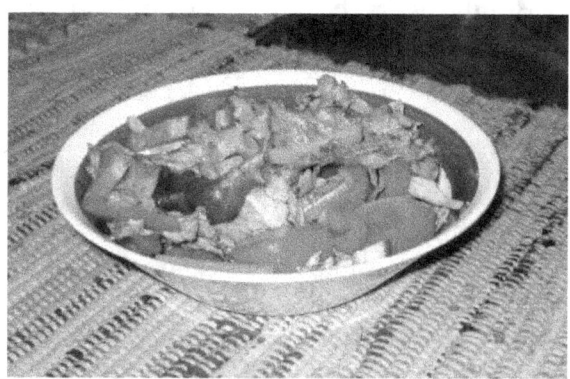

Big-Bowl Salad

Top your "Big-Bowl" with 2 tablespoons of any light salad dressing available at your local supermarket that contains no more than 25 Calories per tablespoon. Some of our favorite light salad dressings are:

- **Ken's Steakhouse Fat Free Raspberry Pecan**
- **Kraft Light Done Right House Italian**
- **Wishbone Just 2 Good Honey Dijon**
- **Newman's Lighten Up! Balsamic Vinaigrette**

Your "Big-Bowl Salad" with two tablespoons of light salad dressing will cost you roughly 150 Calories but will be packed with lots of health-giving vitamins, minerals and fiber.

Snack Guidelines

Most of the menus in the *7-Day No-Cooking Diets* feature a morning snack, an afternoon snack and an evening snack. The main snacks are:

Non-fat Yogurt: Whatever brand you buy be sure to only eat 60 Calories of yogurt for your snack. (Shopping hint: Buy a large 32 oz container of non-fat yogurt, any flavor, and scoop out about 4 oz.)

Fresh Fruit in season: Choose an apple, pear, peach, plum, watermelon (1 cup), etc. You will be eating fruit every day. So vary the fruit that you select to get good array of micronutrients.

Handful of Unsalted Mixed Nuts: Nuts and seeds are loaded with protein and fiber. This book uses a "handful" as a convenient descriptor rather than something like "16 almonds = 100 Calories," but be aware that although nuts are a healthy food, nuts are also a high-calorie food. Buy mixed nuts to get a range of micronutrients. And please no salt.

Skinny Cow Ice Cream Sandwich: This is a relatively low-calorie, low fat, yummy dairy-sweet snack.

Kashi TLC Chewy Granola Bar: A sweet treat packed with whole grains, nuts and seeds. The bar comes in four flavors – with each containing about 140 Calories.

Nabisco 100 Calorie Pack Cookies: A few of Nabisco's popular cookies in a portion controlled 100-Calorie package.

Popcorn Mini Bag: Popcorn is a tasty, nutritious high-fiber, filling snack. For a busy adult consider Orville Redenbacher's Smart Pop Popcorn Mini Bag which you can just nuke and eat. But for the best popcorn we suggest you purchase a hot-air popper which uses popping corn, a type of corn that bursts from the kernel and puffs up when heated. A hot-air popper will make a large batch of popcorn in a few minutes. For a snack, eat only 5 or 6 cups of the popcorn and store the remainder for another day. At this writing, you can buy a hot-air popper for about $25.00.

About Bread

First understand that bread, more specifically whole-grain breads, are good sources of complex carbohydrates and dietary fiber, as well as several B vitamins (thiamin, riboflavin, niacin, and folate), vitamin E, and minerals (iron, magnesium and selenium).

In recent years, however, sliced bread loaves have gotten larger, as have the bread slices inside these loaves. Just a few years ago the standard slice of bread contained about 70 Calories – now most are 100 plus Calories. **The *7-Day No-Cooking Diet* requires whole-grain bread at 70 Calories per slice.** Quite a few bakers sell thin sliced or "light" sliced bread. The difficult part is finding a whole grain thin sliced or "light" bread (with about 70 Calories per slice). Whatever the brand, make sure the first word in the Ingredients list is "whole." "Pepperidge Farm Small Slice 100% Whole Wheat" is a good choice. It's whole grain, has 70 Calories per slice and it tastes good too.

7-Day Diet Facts

The 1,200 and 1,500 Calorie diets adhere to the United States Department of Agriculture recommendation that suggest a balanced diet should have approximately 50 percent of its calories from carbs, about 20 percent from protein sources and 30 percent or less from fat. (Note, the *7-Day No-Cooking Diet* may not be appropriate for individuals with illnesses such as heart disease, diabetes, food allergies, etc. Again, please see your physician before starting any diet.)

<u>900-Calorie Diet:</u> Because of the very low calorie level, this diet does not provide all the nutrients and micro nutrients you need for good health. But over the short term this should not be a problem for healthy adults. Also note that on 900 Calories per day you will undoubtedly feel hungry at times.

<u>1200-Calorie Diet:</u> Due to the relatively low calorie level, you will just barely get all the nutrients and micro nutrients you need – and you also might occasionally feel hungry.

<u>1500 Calorie Diet:</u> This is a reasonable diet calorie level where most adults easily get all the nutrients and micro nutrients they need – and rarely feel hungry.

Important Notes

1) Coffee or tea may be regular or decaf. If desired, skim milk and a sugar substitute may be added to coffee or tea. And soy or almond milk are acceptable substitutes for cow's milk.

2) Fried eggs or scrambled eggs should be cooked in a pan coated with a non-stick cooking spray. Hard-boiled eggs may be substituted for fried, scrambled or soft-boiled eggs.

3) Cereals should be whole grain and unsweetened. At the top of the list are Old-fashioned Oatmeal, Wheatena and Shredded Wheat. Among other reasonably healthy choices are Cheerios, Wheat Chex, Wheaties, some Kashi cereals and Farina. When blueberries are in season, you may add **blueberries instead of raisins** to your cereal. (Substitution ratio = 2 blueberries per raisin.)

4) Bread may be either plain or toasted whole grain, such as whole wheat, whole rye or pumpernickel. Look for whole grain varieties that contain 70 Calories per slice. If desired, bread may be sprayed with a zero-calorie butter substitute.

5) When soup in a microwaveable bowl is specified, eat only one serving (8 ounces) unless otherwise noted. (Microwaveable bowls usually contain about two servings.)

6) Use freely as desired: clear unsweetened coffee, clear unsweetened tea, water, seltzer water and any diet soda, clear soups without fat, bouillon, and seasonings such as mustard, cinnamon, dill, herbs, red and black pepper, curry, vinegar, lemon juice and sections, and dill and sour pickles.

7) Use only lean cuts of meat trimmed of all visible fat. Poultry should be limited to chicken or turkey breasts (white meat only and skinless).

8) When canned tuna or salmon is specified, use only fish packed in water.

9) When the diet calls for turkey bacon, make sure the brand you buy has no more than 35 Calories per slice.

10) An unlimited amount of green salad may be eaten, but the salad dressing should be as specified.

11) Use freely as desired: clear unsweetened coffee, clear unsweetened tea, water, seltzer, any diet soda, clear soups without fat, bouillon, and seasonings such as mustard, cinnamon, dill, herbs, red and black pepper, curry, vinegar, lemon juice and sections, and dill and sour pickles.

12) If it's more convenient, any food item may be moved to any part of the day and combined with any meal or snack.

13) If you cannot find the exact item called for in the diet (because it's out of stock or discontinued), substitute a comparable food (of the same type and close caloric value).

Keeping It Off

Within five years, more than 90 percent of all dieters regain every pound they have lost. Why? In most cases it's because after losing weight most people eventually revert to their pre-diet eating and exercising habits, and this inevitably leads to their regaining the weight they lost– and often more.

The fact is the less you weigh, the less you need to eat to sustain your lower weight.

A study, published in the Annals of Internal Medicine that followed 4,000 people for three decades suggests that in the long term, 90 percent of men and 70 percent of women will become overweight. Interestingly, half of the men and women in the study, who had made it well into adulthood without a weight problem, ultimately also became overweight and a third actually became obese. The point being that you can never become complacent. You must continually watch your weight because we are all at risk of becoming overweight.

As mentioned previously, the key to long-term weight control success is knowledge and understanding, combined of course with desire and self-discipline. Once more, for the full story see *Weight Control - U.S. Edition* by Vincent Antonetti, Ph.D., or *Weight Maintenance - U.S. Edition* also by Vincent Antonetti, both published by NoPaperPress.com.

Appendix C
Soup Selections

When the Daily Meal Plan menu specifies soup have only one serving (8 ounces) unless stated otherwise. Note that the listed soups were available in most supermarkets as of 02/14/2020. *These are a canned soup selections.

Soup Description	Calories
Healthy Choice Chicken with Rice	90
Campbell's Tomato	100
Healthy Choice Country Vegetable	100
Progresso Minestrone*	110
Progresso Chickarina*	110
Progresso Italian-Style Wedding*	120
Campbell's Home-Style Light Chicken Corn Chowder*	120
Campbell's Home-Style Chicken Noodle	130
Campbell's Home-Style Butter Nut Squash*	130
Campbell's Healthy Request Vegetable Beef	140
Progresso Lentil*	140
Progresso Green Split Pea*	150
Campbell's Slow Kettle New England Clam Chowder	160
Progresso Macaroni and Bean*	160
Progresso New England Clam Chowder*	170
Progresso Lasagna-Style*	170
Progresso Broccoli Cheese with Bacon*	180
As an alternative, have 2 servings of a 90 Cal soup	180
Campbell's Chunky Classic Chicken Noodle	190
Amy's Rustic Italian Vegetable*	190
Campbell's Chunky Beef n Cheese*	200
Amy's French Country Vegetable*	210
Campbell's Chunky Sirloin Burger + Vegetables	220
Enjoy two servings of a 110 or 120 Calorie soup	230
Enjoy two servings of a 120 Calorie soup	240

Appendix D
Frozen Entrées

Appendix D lists three popular brands of frozen entrées: Healthy Choice, Lean Cuisine and Smart Ones. Note that each brand is color coded. The listing is further divided by entrée type: Poultry entrées, Meat entrées, Seafood entrées, Pasta entrées, Pizza and Other entrées. The entire table is arranged from the lowest to highest in calories. Note that the listed frozen entrées were available in most super markets as of 02/14/2020.

Type	Name	Brand	Calories
Poultry	Tomato Basil Chicken & Spinach	Smart Ones	160
Meat	Steak Portobella	Lean Cuisine	160
Meat	Asian Style Beef & Broccoli	Smart Ones	~~160~~ 170
Poultry	Herb Roasted Chicken	Lean Cuisine	170
Poultry	Slow Roasted Turkey Breast	Smart Ones	170
Poultry	Grilled Chicken Marsala	Healthy Choice	180
Poultry	Creamy Basil Chicken w Broccoli	Smart Ones	~~180~~ 170
Poultry	Garlic Chicken Rolls	Lean Cuisine	180
Meat	Beef Merlot	Healthy Choice	180
Meat	Homestyle Beef Pot Roast	Smart Ones	180
Poultry	Roasted Turkey & Vegetables	Lean Cuisine	190
Poultry	Chicken & Broccoli Alfredo	Healthy Choice	190
Poultry	Chicken & Vegetable Stir Fry	Healthy Choice	190
Other	Broccoli & Cheddar Roast Potato	Smart Ones	190
Poultry	Crustless Chicken Pot Pie	Smart Ones	~~200~~ 190
Poultry	Buffalo Style Chicken	Lean Cuisine	~~200~~ 190
Poultry	Home Style Chicken & Potatoes	Healthy Choice	200
Pasta	Angel Hair Marinara	Smart Ones	200
Poultry	Salisbury Steak	Smart Ones	200
Meat	Roast Beef & Mashed Potatoes	Smart Ones	~~220~~ 200
Pasta	Primavera Pasta	Smart Ones	210

Poultry	Honey Balsamic Chicken	Healthy Choice	210
Pasta	Ravioli Florentine	Smart Ones	210
Poultry	Cajun Style Chicken & Shrimp	Healthy Choice	220
Pasta	Cheese Ravioli Mushroom Sauce	Smart Ones	230
Poultry	Ranchero Chicken Wrap	Smart Ones	230
Poultry	Lemon Herb Chicken Picante	Smart Ones	230
Pasta	Cheese Ravioli Mushroom Sauce	Smart Ones	230
Meat	Meat Loaf with Mashed Potatoes	Lean Cuisine	~~230~~ 240
Seafood	Shrimp Alfredo	Lean Cuisine	~~230~~ 240
Poultry	Chicken Margherita	Smart Ones	~~220~~ 240
Poultry	Grilled Chicken Caesar	Lean Cuisine	240
Poultry	Honey Glazed Turkey & Potatoes	Healthy Choice	240
Pasta	Spicy Penne Arrabbiata	Lean Cuisine	240
Pasta	Four Cheese Cannelloni	Lean Cuisine	~~240~~ 250
Poultry	Creamy Basil Chicken w Tortellini	Lean Cuisine	~~240~~ 250
Pasta	Cheese Ravioli	Lean Cuisine	250
Pasta	Vermont Cheddar Mac & Cheese	Lean Cuisine	250
Pasta	Fettuccini Alfredo	Smart Ones	250
Poultry	Oriental Chicken	Smart Ones	250
Poultry	Fiesta Grilled Chicken	Lean Cuisine	250
Pasta	Chicken Linguini Red Pepper	Healthy Choice	250
Poultry	Golden Roasted Turkey Breast	Healthy Choice	250
Poultry	Chicken Mesquite	Smart Ones	250
Poultry	Chicken Oriental	Smart Ones	250
Poultry	Orange Sesame Chicken	Smart Ones	250
Poultry	Baked Chicken	Lean Cuisine	~~250~~ 260
Poultry	Teriyaki Chicken & Vegetables	Smart Ones	~~250~~ 260
Seafood	Tuna Noodle Casserole	Smart Ones	~~250~~ 270
Pasta	Spaghetti with Meatballs	Lean Cuisine	260
Poultry	Creamy Chicken & Noodles	Healthy Choice	260

Meat	Barbecue Steak w Red Potatoes	Healthy Choice	260
Pasta	Tortellini Primavera Parmesan	Healthy Choice	260
Pasta	Sesame Noodles with Vegetables	Smart Ones	260 280
Pasta	Creamy Rigatoni w Chicken	Smart Ones	260
Pasta	Macaroni & Cheese	Smart Ones	260
Pasta	Butternut Squash Ravioli	Lean Cuisine	260
Other	Santa Fe Rice & Beans	Smart Ones	260
Other	Coconut Chickpea Curry	Lean Cuisine	260
Poultry	Glazed Turkey Tenderloins	Lean Cuisine	270
Poultry	Kung Pao Chicken	Healthy Choice	270
Poultry	Chicken Margherita w Balsamic	Healthy Choice	270
Poultry	Chicken Strips & Sweet Potatoes	Smart Ones	270
Pasta	Spaghetti with Meat Sauce	Smart Ones	270 280
Meat	Salisbury Steak with Mac & Cheese	Lean Cuisine	270 290
Pasta	Penne Rosa	Lean Cuisine	270
Poultry	Turkey Breast & Stuffing	Smart Ones	270 280
Pasta	Classic Macaroni & Beef	Lean Cuisine	270
Pasta	Mushroom Mezzaluna Ravioli	Lean Cuisine	270
Pasta	Pasta with Swedish Meatballs	Smart Ones	280 290
Other	Asian Pot Stickers	Lean Cuisine	280
Poultry	Sesame Stir Fry with Chicken	Lean Cuisine	280
Poultry	Roasted Turkey Breast	Lean Cuisine	280 290
Poultry	Apple Cranberry Chicken	Lean Cuisine	280
Poultry	Chicken Fettuccini Alfredo	Healthy Choice	280
Poultry	Grilled Chicken Marinara	Healthy Choice	280
Poultry	Sweet & Spicy Orange Chicken	Healthy Choice	280
Poultry	Chicken Parmesan	Smart Ones	280
Poultry	Turkey Breast with Stuffing	Smart Ones	280
Meat	Beef & Broccoli	Healthy Choice	280
Meat	Meatball Marinara	Healthy Choice	280

Meat	Beef Teriyaki	Healthy Choice	280
Pasta	Spinach Artichoke Ravioli	Lean Cuisine	280
Other	Vegetable Fried Rice	Smart Ones	280
Pasta	Spinach Artichoke Ravioli	Lean Cuisine	280
Pasta	Linguini with Ricotta & Spinach	Lean Cuisine	280
Poultry	Chicken Fettuccini	Lean Cuisine	~~290~~ 280
Pasta	Spaghetti & Meatballs	Healthy Choice	280
Pasta	Spaghetti with Meat Sauce	Smart Ones	280
Other	Vegetable Fried Rice	Smart Ones	280
Other	Asian Pot Stickers	Lean Cuisine	280
Poultry	Chicken with Almonds	Lean Cuisine	290
Poultry	Chicken with Peanut Sauce	Lean Cuisine	290
Seafood	Shrimp & Angel Hair Pasta	Lean Cuisine	~~280~~ 290
Poultry	Grilled Chicken Pesto w Veggies	Healthy Choice	290
Poultry	General Tso's Spicy Chicken	Healthy Choice	290
Poultry	Pineapple Chicken	Healthy Choice	290
Poultry	Chicken Enchiladas Suiza	Smart Ones	290
Meat	Swedish Meatballs	Lean Cuisine	290
Seafood	Lemon Pepper Fish	Healthy Choice	290
Pasta	Pasta with Swedish Meatballs	Smart Ones	290
Other	Santa Fe Rice & Beans	Smart Ones	290
Pizza	Thin Crust Cheese Pizza	Smart Ones	290
Seafood	Parmesan Crusted Fish	Lean Cuisine	~~290~~ 300
Pasta	Santa Fe-Style Rice & Beans	Lean Cuisine	~~280~~ 300
Poultry	Roasted Turkey & Vegetables	Lean Cuisine	~~290~~ 300
Poultry	Sweet & Sour Chicken	Lean Cuisine	300
Poultry	Crustless Chicken Pot Pie	Healthy Choice	300
Poultry	Sweet Sesame Chicken	Healthy Choice	300
Poultry	Chicken Fettuccini	Smart Ones	300
Poultry	General Tso's Chicken	Smart Ones	300

Meat	Classic Meat Loaf	Healthy Choice	300
Seafood	Tortilla Crusted Fish	Lean Cuisine	~~300~~ 310
Pasta	Tuscan-Style Vegetable Lasagna	Lean Cuisine	~~300~~ 310
Pasta	Tortellini with Red Pepper Sauce	Lean Cuisine	300
Pasta	Broccoli Cheddar Rotini	Lean Cuisine	300
Pasta	Three Cheese Ziti Marinara	Smart Ones	300
Pasta	Lasagna Florentine	Smart Ones	~~310~~ 300
Seafood	Tortilla Crusted Fish	Lean Cuisine	~~300~~ 310
Pasta	Tuscan-Style Vegetable Lasagna	Lean Cuisine	~~300~~ 310
Poultry	Chicken Fried Rice	Lean Cuisine	~~300~~ 310
Poultry	Orange Chicken	Lean Cuisine	310
Poultry	Chicken Tikka Masala	Lean Cuisine	310
Poultry	Chicken Strips & Fries	Smart Ones	310
Poultry	Chicken Teriyaki	Lean Cuisine	310
Pizza	Thin Crust Pepperoni Pizza	Smart Ones	310
Pasta	Three Cheese Macaroni	Smart Ones	310
Pizza	French Bread Pepperoni Pizza	Lean Cuisine	310
Poultry	Chicken Spinach Mushroom Panini	Lean Cuisine	~~350~~ 310
Other	Spicy Beef & Bean Enchilada	Lean Cuisine	310
Poultry	Chicken Fried Rice	Healthy Choice	320
Meat	Sweet & Spicy Korean Beef	Lean Cuisine	320
Pizza	Farmers Market Pizza	Lean Cuisine	320
Pizza	Margherita Pizza	Lean Cuisine	320
Poultry	Chicken Carbonara	Lean Cuisine	330
Poultry	Mango Chicken w Coconut Rice	Lean Cuisine	330
Poultry	Country Fried Chicken	Healthy Choice	330
Other	Cheese & Fire-Roasted Tamale	Lean Cuisine	330
Poultry	Chicken Club Panini	Lean Cuisine	~~350~~ 340
Meat	Philly Style Steak & Cheese Panini	Lean Cuisine	~~330~~ 350
Poultry	Chicken Parmigiana	Healthy Choice	360

Appendix E
Frozen Food Safety

Increasingly, food giants like ConAgra, Nestlé and others that supply Americans with processed foods concede that they cannot ensure the safety of their food products. Frozen foods pose a particularly serious safety problem because unsuspecting consumers buy frozen foods for their convenience and incorrectly believe that cooking frozen foods is a matter of taste – not safety.

Still the food industry says that extensive outbreaks of food-borne illness are rare, even though it is well-known that most of the millions of cases of food-borne illness every year go unreported or are not traced to the source. For example, each year approximately 40,000 cases of salmonella poisoning are reported in the United States – but perhaps as many as one million cases go unreported. (Salmonella is a type of bacteria most often found in poultry, eggs, unprocessed milk, meat and water.) Recently salmonella pathogens in some frozen meals have sickened thousands of people. How could this happen? First, the supply chain for ingredients in processed foods – from flour to fruits and vegetables to flavorings – is becoming more complex and global in the drive to keep food costs down. As a result, government and industry officials concede that almost every food ingredient is now a potential carrier of pathogens. A further complication is that a large number of food companies subcontract processing work to save money and don't require suppliers to test for pathogens. In fact, companies often don't even know who is supplying their ingredients.

In addition, many frozen-food manufacturers have stopped cooking their products at high temperatures, a tactic they call the "kill step," which is intended to eliminate any lingering microbes. Frequently this process step turns some of the frozen food ingredients into mush. So, instead the "kill step" has been shifted to consumers. For example, ConAgra has added food safety instructions to its frozen meals, including the Healthy Choice brand. A typical "frozen-food safety" instruction offers this guidance: "Internal temperature needs to reach 165°F as measured by a food thermometer in several spots." Moreover, General Mills, now advises consumers to avoid microwaves altogether and cook frozen pizzas in a conventional oven. **Bottom line**: To be safe, always cook frozen foods so that the internal temperature reaches 165°F as measured by a good food thermometer.

100-Day Super Diet-1200 Calorie*	Weight Loss for Men - Metric*
100-Day Super Diet-1500 Calorie*	Maximum Weight Loss- 1200 Calorie*
100-Day No-Cooking Diet-1200 Cal*	Maximum Weight Loss- 1500 Calorie*
100-Day No-Cooking Diet-1500 Cal*	Weight Control - U.S. Edition
90-Day Smart Diet-1200 Calorie*	Weight Control - Metric. Edition
90-Day Smart Diet-1500 Calorie*	Professional Weight Control Women - U.S.
90-Day No-Cooking Diet - 1200 Cal*	Professional Weight Control Women - Metric
90-Day No-Cooking Diet - 1500 Cal*	Professional Weight Control Men - U.S.
90-Day Perfect Diet - 1200 Calorie*	Professional Weight Control Men - Metric
90-Day Perfect Diet - 1500 Calorie*	Weight Maintenance - U.S. Edition*
60-Day Perfect Diet-1200 Calorie*	Weight Maintenance - Metric. Edition*
60-Day Perfect Diet-1500 Calorie*	Weight Maintenance - UK Edition
50-Day Flex Diet-1200 Calorie*	Weight Loss for Senior Men*
50-Day Flex Diet-1500 Calorie*	Weight Loss for Senior Women*
30-Day Quick Diet - for Women*	Eat Smart - U.S. Edition*
30-Day Quick Diet - for Men*	Eat Smart - Metric Edition
30-Day No-Cooking Diet*	30-Day Mediterranean Diet
30-Day Diet for Women - Metric*	Exercise Smart - U.S. Edition*
30-Day Diet for Men - Metric*	Exercise Smart - Metric Edition
25 Day Easy Diet-1200 Calorie*	Exercise Smart - UK Edition*
25 Day Easy Diet-1500 Calorie*	Total Fitness - U.S. Edition
25-Day No-Cooking Diet	Total Fitness - Metric Edition
10-Day Express Diet	Total Fitness - UK Edition
10-Day No-Cooking Diet*	Total Fitness for Women-U.S. Edition*
7-Day Diet for Women*	Total Fitness for Women - Metric
7-Day Diet for Men*	Total Fitness for Women - UK Edition
7-Day No-Cooking Diets*	Total Fitness for Men - U.S. Edition*
90-Day Gluten-Free Diet-1200 Cal*	Total Fitness for Men- Metric Edition*
90-Day Gluten-Free Diet-1500 Cal*	Total Fitness for Men - UK Edition
30-Day Gluten-Free Quick Diet*	Senior Fitness - U.S. Edition*
30-Day Gluten-Free No-Cooking Diet*	Senior Fitness - Metric Edition*
7-Day Diet for Women - Metric*	Senior Fitness - UK Edition*
7-Day Diet for Men - Metric	Computer Diet - U.S. Edition*
7-Day Gluten-Free Express Diet*	Computer Diet - Metric Edition*
7-Day Gluten-Free No-Cooking Diet*	Reliable Weight Loss - U.S. Edition
90-Day Vegetarian Diet-1200 Calorie*	101 Weight Loss Tips*
90-Day Vegetarian Diet-1500 Calorie*	101 Healthy Eating Tips*
30-Day Vegetarian Diet*	101 Lifelong Fitness Tips*
7-Day Vegetarian Diet*	101 Weight Maintenance Tips
Weight Loss for Women*	101 Weight Loss Recipes
Weight Loss for Women - Metric	101 Gluten-Free Weight Loss Recipes
Weight Loss for Women - UK	101 Vegetarian Weight Loss Recipes*
Weight Loss for Men*	30-Day Mediterranean Diet*
Maximum Weight Loss - 1200 Cal*	90-Day Mediterranean Diet - 1200 Cal*
Maximum Weight Loss - 1500 Cal*	90-Day Mediterranean Diet - 1500 Cal*

* These titles are available as both ebooks and paperbacks. Our ebooks are sold by Amazon, Apple, Google, Barnes & Noble and Kobo. But paperbacks are only sold by Amazon.

Disclaimer

This book offers general meal planning, nutrition and weight control information. It is not a medical manual and the author does not claim to be medically qualified. The material in this book is not intended to be a substitute for medical counseling. Everyone should have a medical checkup before beginning a weight loss program. Moreover, the physician conducting the medical exam should be made aware of and should approve the specific weight control program planned. Additionally, while the author and publisher have made every effort to ensure the accuracy of the information in this book, they make no representations or warranties regarding its accuracy or completeness. Further, neither the author nor publisher assume liability for any medical problems that might result from applying the methods in this book, or for any loss of profit, or any other commercial damages, including but not limited to special, incidental, consequential or other damages, and any such liability is hereby expressly disclaimed.